OKOMI
Wanders Too Far

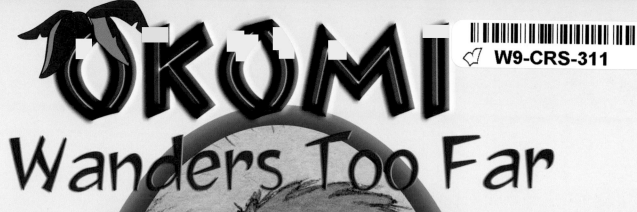

Helen and
Clive Dorman

Illustrated by
Tony Hutchings

Dawn Publications
in association with The Jane Goodall Institute

Okomi and his mommy,
Mama Du, were walking
in the forest. It had just stopped
raining and the air felt fresh.

Mama Du was taking Okomi
to search for fruit.

She took him down
a path he did not know.

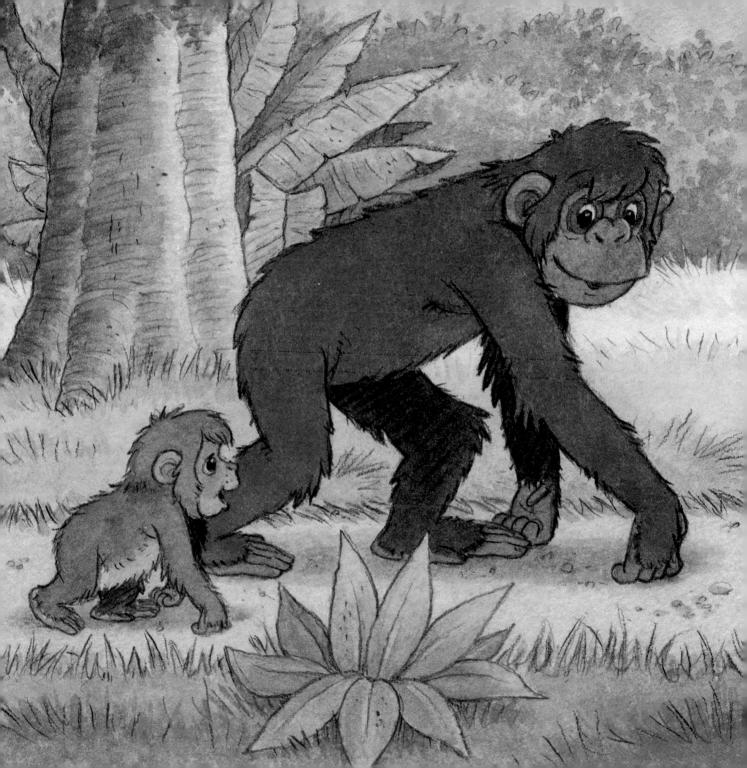

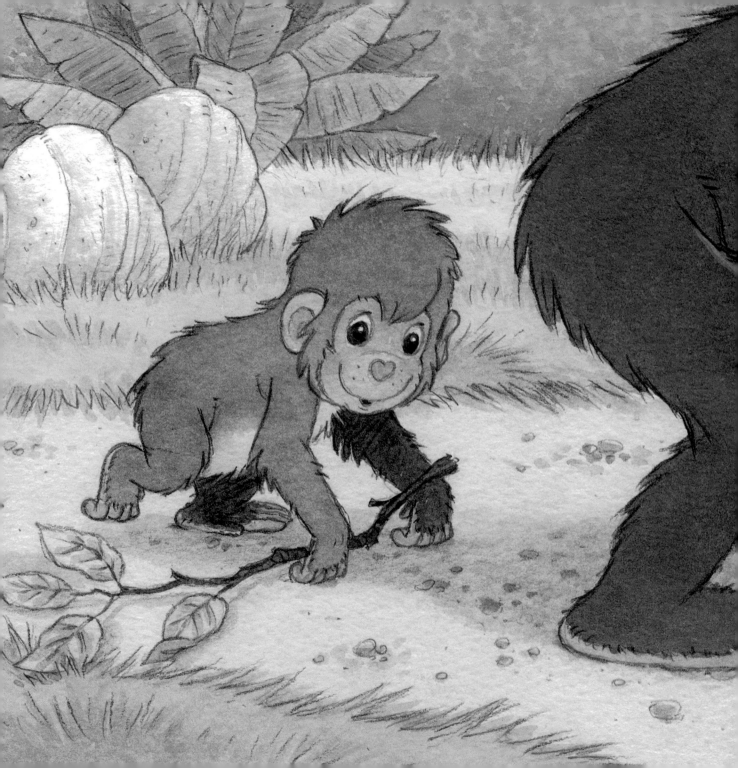

Okomi was excited.
He loved new places
to explore.

Okomi found a leafy branch
and was busy dragging it
along the ground.

He did not notice that
Mama Du had stopped
ahead of him.

Bump! Oops!

Okomi walked right into
his mommy. Mama Du
grunted loudly.

There were two paths ahead, one
on the right and one on the left.
Mama Du wandered up the right
hand path.

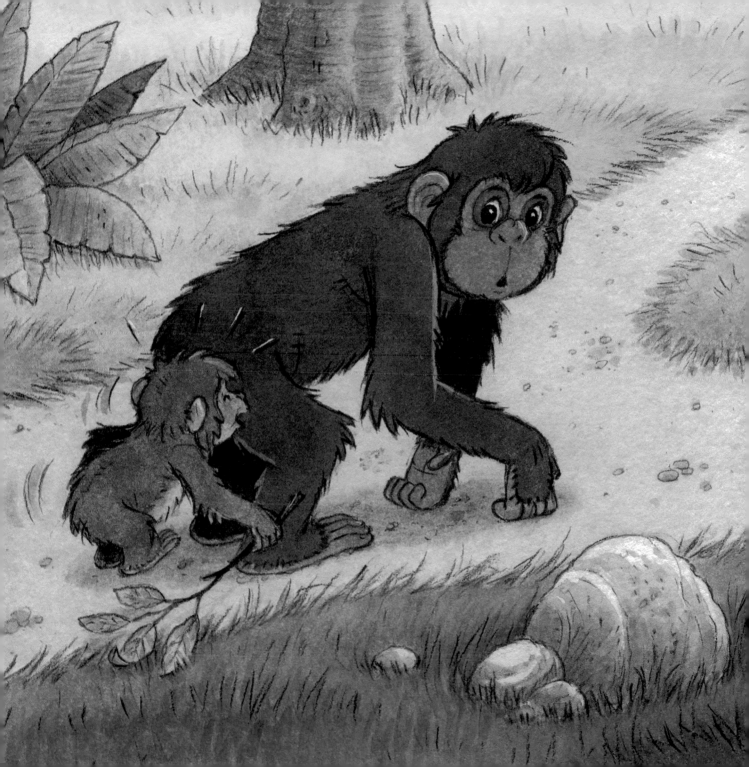

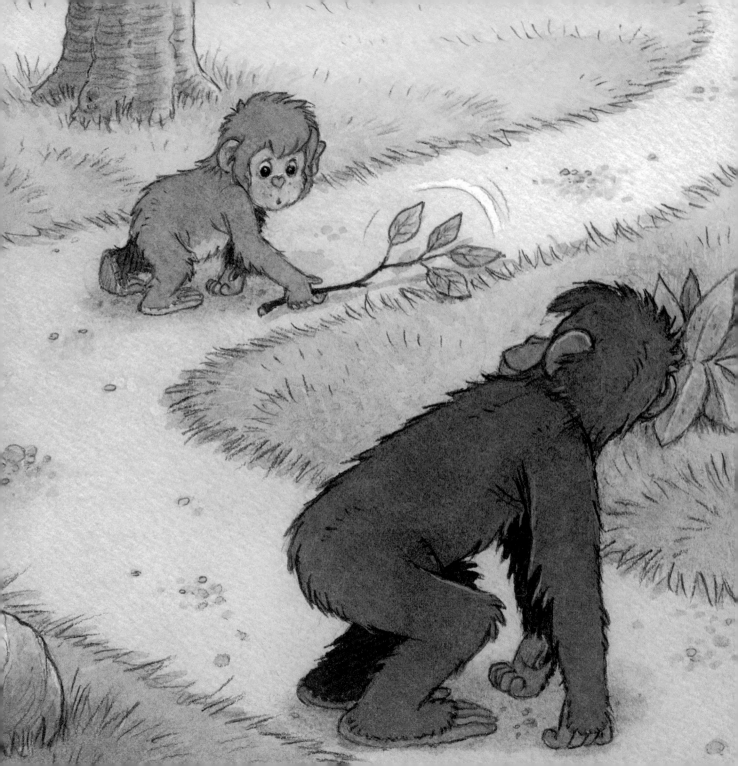

Okomi wanted to go along the other path. He began to whimper and shake the leafy branch to get his mommy's attention. He wanted her to follow him.

Mama Du looked round, waited and then continued up the right hand path.

Okomi whimpered louder.

He went a bit further up
his path and paused to see if
Mama Du was following him.

But she was not.

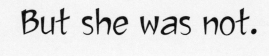

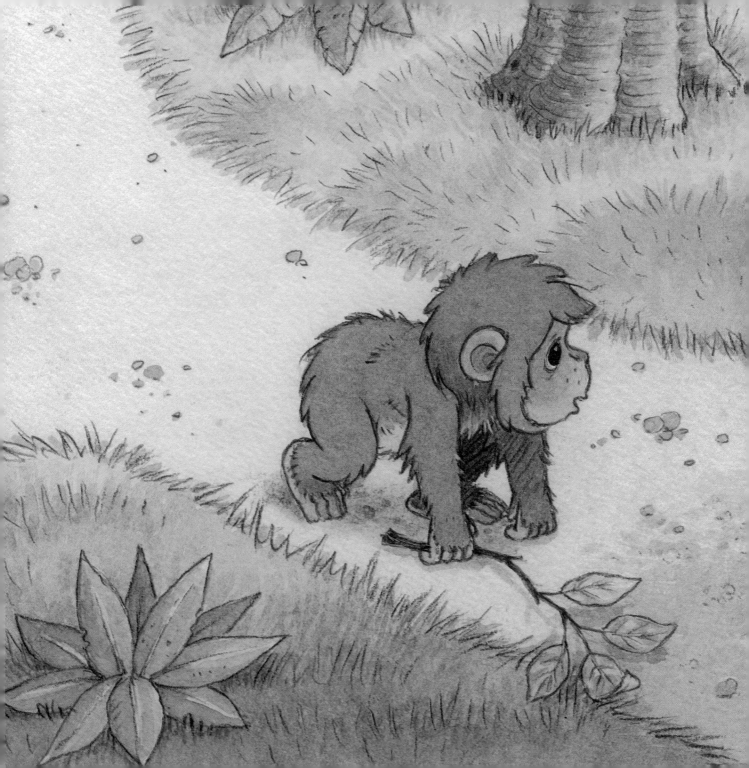

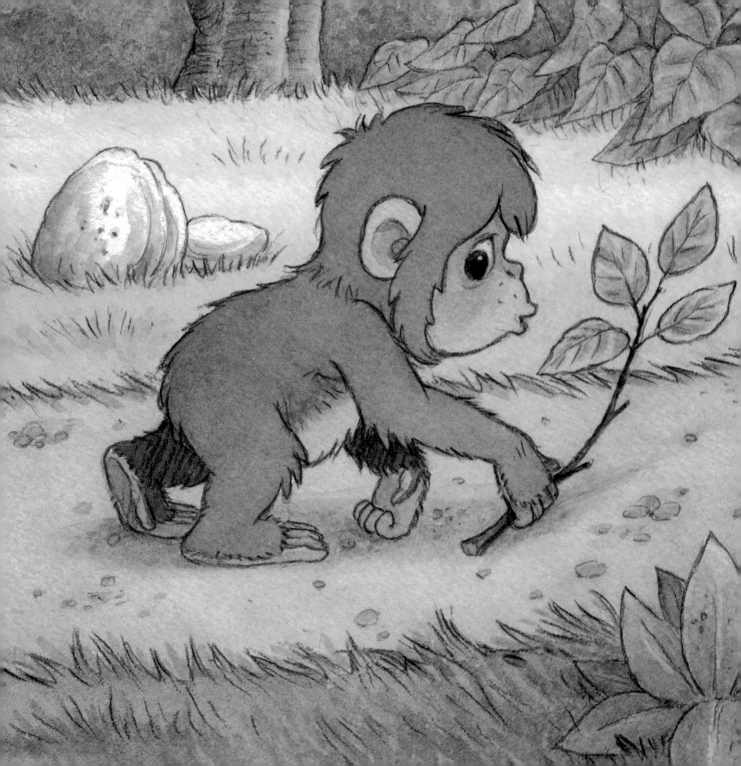

Okomi cried out loud.
He was becoming worried.

If he went any further
he would be out of sight
of his mommy.

Then Okomi heard a rustling
sound coming from some
tall grass nearby.

He stopped still.

What could it be?

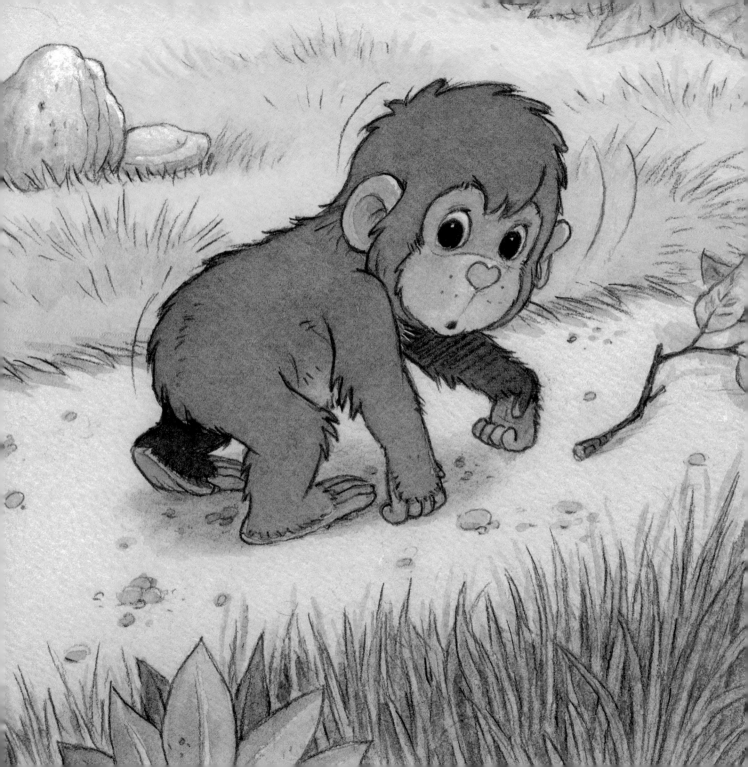

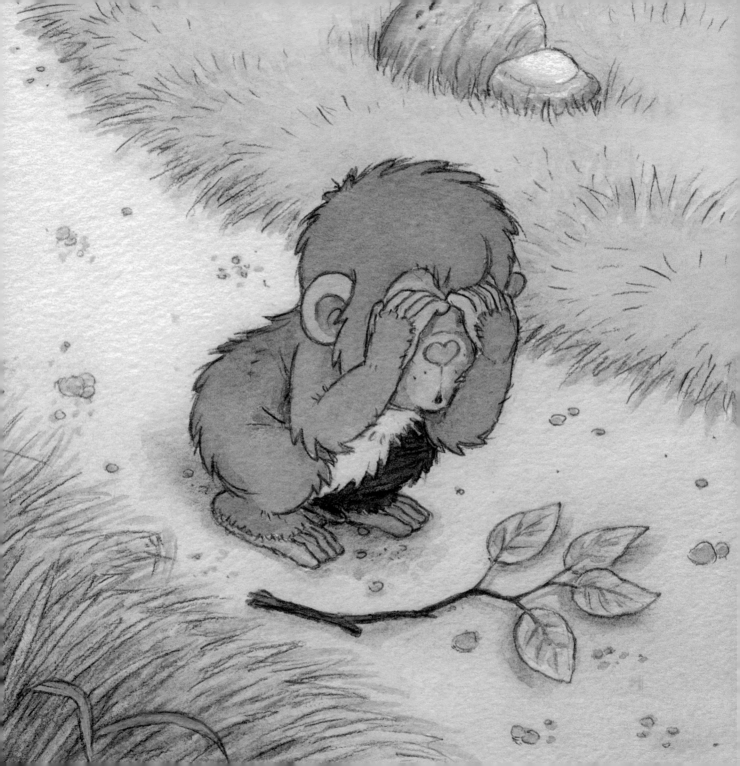

Okomi was frightened.

He did not dare to look.

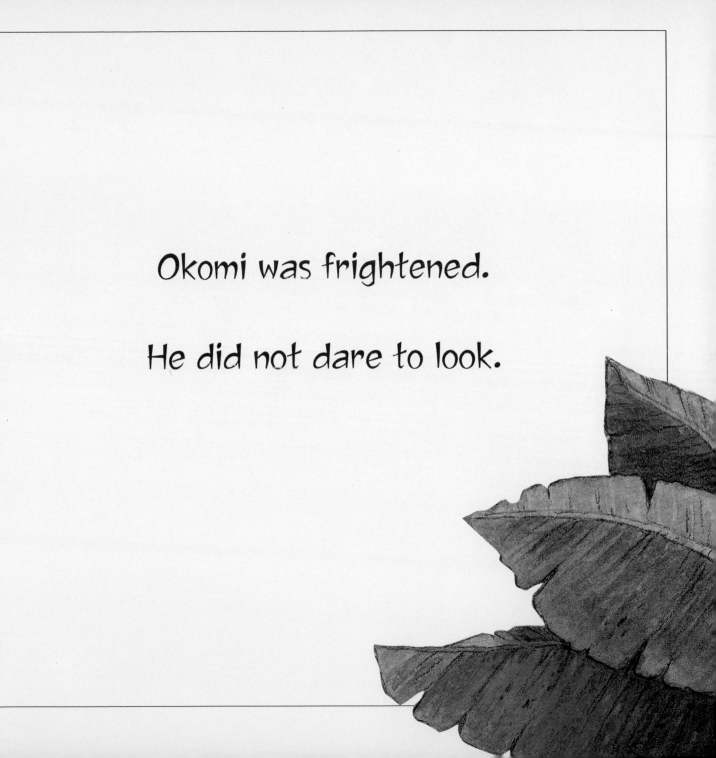

Suddenly, three baby
porcupines ran noisily out
from the tall grass.

Okomi shrieked with fear.

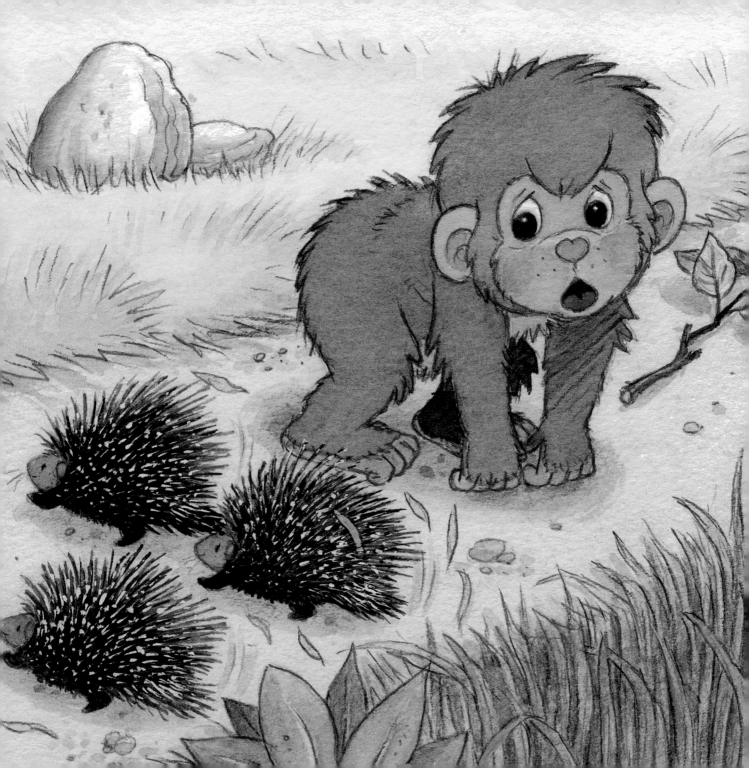

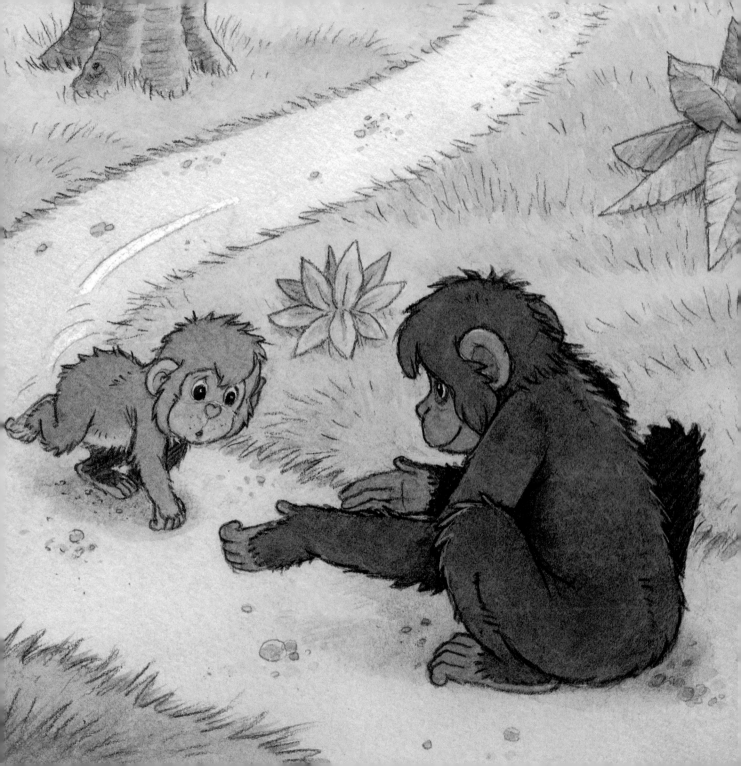

Okomi ran as fast as he could
back along the forest path
to where Mama Du
was waiting for him.

Phew!

He was very pleased
to see his mommy.

Mama Du gave Okomi
a big hug and lifted him on
to her back to safety.

She wandered off down the
right hand path to forage
for fruit.

Mama Du was right after all!

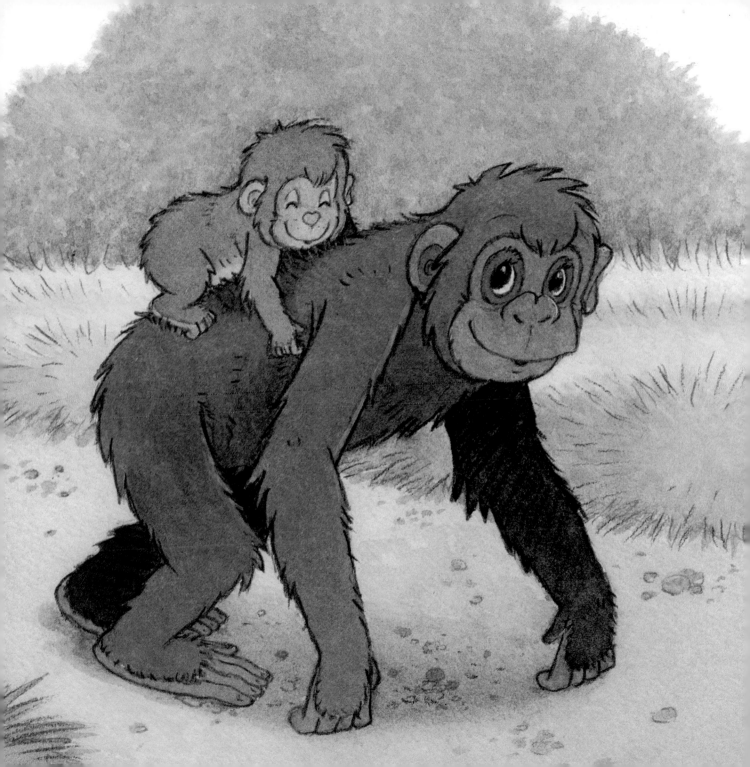

Did you know?

Chimpanzees love to hug and kiss their friends and family. There are close bonds between family members. They are very intelligent.

When they are very young, baby chimpanzees cling to their mother's tummy. When they are about six months old, baby chimpanzees start to ride on their mother's back. At about the same age they start learning to walk and to climb trees.

Young chimps remain with their mothers until they are seven or eight years old. Chimpanzees in the wild can live for as long as 50 years.

Chimpanzees are our closest living relatives in the animal kingdom. These apes are found in the wild only in Africa. They share over 98% of their genetic material with us; they use and make tools; they express many of the same emotions that we do.

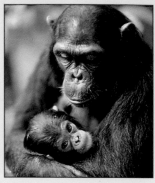

Fanni and her baby, Fax

Helping orphaned chimps

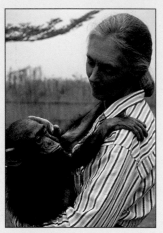

Jane with an orphan chimpanzee

Sadly, chimpanzee numbers are falling as their forests are cut down and they are hunted for the commercial bushmeat trade. This leaves hundreds of orphan chimps. An orphan chimpanzee can almost never be returned to the wild. Proceeds from the sale of each Okomi book supports the Tchimpounga sanctuary (in the Republic of Congo), where there are currently over 100 orphan chimps.

Roots & Shoots

One day in 1991, 16 students gathered on Dr. Jane Goodall's front porch in Dar es Salaam, Tanzania. They were fascinated by animal behavior and environmental concerns, but none of their classes covered these topics. They wanted to know how to help chimpanzees and other animals. Those 16 students went back to their schools to form clubs with other interested young people, and Roots & Shoots began. Since then, the program has spread rapidly throughout the world. More than 3,000 Roots & Shoots groups for children pre-K and up have formed in more than 68 countries around the world. There are many active groups in the U.S. and Canada.

Their mission is to foster respect and compassion for all living things, to promote understanding of all cultures and beliefs and to inspire each individual to take action to make the world a better place for the environment, animals and the human community. For more information contact the Jane Goodall Institute, P.O. Box 14890, Silver Spring, MD 20910, or call (301) 565-0086, or go to www.janegoodall.org.

Dawn Publications is dedicated to inspiring in children a deeper understanding and appreciation for all life on Earth. To view our full list of titles, or to order, please visit our web site at www.dawnpub.com, or call 800-545-7475.